Guide to How to Resist Smoking cigarettes and Quit for Good

Robert R.Gonzales

Table of contents

Chapter 1

Illicit drug use is a constant focal sensory system issue and one of the most serious general medical issues worldwide, not just as a result of their high commonness and effect on the individual, family, work-related and social circles, but yet additionally in light of their monetary and clinical outcomes. The most conspicuous highlight of habit-forming conduct is desiring which can be depicted as the clairvoyant torment of enslavement. It is an obstinate hindrance defied by junkies endeavoring to accomplish forbearance. Hankering is the key to advancing medication bringing conduct into an urgent medication taking a way of behaving. Desires for food are like substance desires in their maladaptive potential to cause dietary issues. The direct connection between hankering and backslide, however not handily settled, seems to happen through moderate variables. Consolidating hankering estimations in routine clinical practice can expand the patient's capacity to be aware of and screen his inner states that are connected with substance admission and this can be utilized in suggesting fitting treatment. Hankering is by all accounts a non-unitary peculiarity, and various types of hankering with various systems have been proposed, so it is possible that various medications can be pretty much successful on various types of hankering. Consequently, there is an incredible requirement for mental administration as an expanded upkeep procedure.

• Strategies that are intended to diminish the probability of the beginning of hankering that incorporate improvement control, signal openness, revolution treatment, adapting symbolism, self-checking, and expertise preparing for staying away from circumstances in which hankering is probably going to happen.

• Systems that are intended to diminish the force and term of hankering that incorporate mental and social ability preparation.

There are various ways of tending to hankering. The ID of triggers or precipitants is the main move toward managing hankering in Persuasive Upgrade Treatment (MET) and Backslide Avoidance Treatment (RPT). Depicted beneath are a couple of well-known ways successful in taking care of hankering utilized in MET and RPT.

• Improvement control: The recurrence of remotely set-off inclinations and hankering can be decreased by utilizing boost control procedures intended to limit openness to the prompts. In certain conditions, keeping away from the circumstance is the best methodology, particularly in those loaded up with various signs of guilty pleasure. This intends that before adapting reactions are solid, certain exercises ought to be reduced until openness to these signs can be dominated without encouraging a pass [1].

• Prompt openness: Sign openness includes redundant openness to signs, a method that is expected to deliver eradication of hankering reactions. Signal openness is best when openness to liquor or medication prompts is matched with procedures and methods intended to plan clients to adapt to the sorts of enticements they will experience throughout their day-to-day existence. Prompt openness medicines have shown viability in diminishing backslide to liquor, nicotine, sedatives, and cocaine [2].

• Revolution treatment: Repugnance treatment includes matching liquor signals with an aversive upgrade, a technique by which liquor prompts come to evoke an aversive response instead of hankering. As opposed to signal openness, the objective of abhorrence treatment is to expand reactivity to liquor prompts, because such sign reactivity is expected to reflect molded sickness. Increment substantial response following aversive response ought to be related to effective results

• Adapting Symbolism: An individual encountering a desire for a substance or movement tends to feel as though the tension is developing inside them and that it will mount sharply until their purpose declines and their opposition falls under the staggering tension of a quickly expanding inflatable that will ultimately detonate. Utilizing a wave illustration created Adapting the Symbolism method, "Urge Surfing", can be utilized to assist the client with overseeing these unmanageable occasions.

• Ask surfing: In this procedure, the client is first educated to name these interior sensations and mental distractions as a desire or hankering that is starting to create and cultivate a demeanor of separation and disrecognizable proof concerning this flood of want. Clients are at first shown the urge riding strategy through directed symbolism and afterward give it a shot on their own at whatever point they are presented with substance prompts. One exhortation that functions admirably in clinical circumstances is that of End, which incorporates the four D's. If one dodges these circumstances, the probability of hankering diminishes

condition

• Self-observing of desires and hankering - The Desire Journal: One more method for encouraging separation from inclinations and hankering is to have clients utilize Self-Checking Systems to follow along on these encounters. The client is approached to monitor the inward and outside signals that invigorate the desire, their mindset, the strength of the hankering, how long it endured, adapting abilities, for example, encourage riding used to adapt to the hankering, and how fruitful or ineffective these ways of dealing with especially difficult times were [1].

• Interactive ability preparing: These incorporate figuring out how to deny like a patient rejecting a genuine glass of brew, subsequently figuring out how to produce a proper reaction under reasonable conditions, others resembling requesting that a companion forego savoring one's presence [3].

• Social procedures: These incorporate utilization of nonalcoholic beverages or food, calling a companion to examine the hankering, getting some actual activity, reading, especially about recuperation, keeping occupied, occupying oneself with an action, staying away from high-risk individuals, spots, and occasions, be firm while denying offers to utilize substances [3].

• Mental systems: These incorporate recalling the result of consuming or not consuming, a reappraisal of the circumstance, recollecting one's obligation to restraint, recollecting that desires and longings for substances, in the end, disappear, thinking positively and letting oneself know that she/he can fend off wanting, talking oneself through the hankering, imploring or requesting strength from a higher power, rehearsing quite a bit early how to deny substance offers3. Mental changes related to sign evoked hankering and intriguing that desire for liquor is trailed by culpability/loss of certainty, alongside feelings which for the most part result from fruitless adapting and backslide. Maybe desiring itself addressed disappointment. These discoveries infer that objective of treatment ought to be to assist patients with seeing desire as typical and view opposing hankering to act as an illustration of fruitful adapting [3]. The desires as a rule don't work at a cognizant level, yet are probably going to be covered by the mental mutilations and safeguard components. Thusly, these faintly seen sensations and compelling feelings loaded up with prohibited wants to set up the chance of backsliding by carrying the individual nearer to openness to a high-risk circumstance. Training patients to become watchful for these early advance notice signals and to take part in express self-talk which questions their inspirations and goals can assist them with perceiving and recognizing the immediate importance of these "Evidently Immaterial Choices" to the expanded gamble of backsliding. This might permit the patient to start to see through their justification and disavowal by perceiving the genuine significance and reasonable result (backslide) of the choices they may not be assuming a sense of ownership in making

Mental conduct treatment in needing

Social methods principally center around an aversion to animating circumstances, a different reaction to these energizers, and offering new proper fortifications. Mental strategies assist patients with perceiving contemplations that go before drug use and supplant them with better considerations. Along these lines, patients figure out how to take a gander at circumstances and relations another way [4].

Pollack et al. (2002) [5] concentrated on the viability of mental conduct treatment on diminishing hankering and proposed that mental conduct treatment manages to assist the patient with perceiving outside and interior energizers and apply powerful techniques. This mediation is likewise powerful in breaking the connection between bad temperament and medication use.

Hankering as metacognition

Understanding desires as metacognition means that the individual is encountering mental occasions, like desultory reasoning, sentiments, recollections, insights, sensations, dreams, or pictures, and evaluates as aversive and wishes to alter as quickly as could be expected. A metacognitive examination of hankering stresses the speed with which medications and liquor can influence emotional experience because the change of cognizant experience is one of the most dependable and mentally significant impacts of psychoactive substances, frequently happening inside the space of seconds or minutes

The four reasons for hankering are recognized:

• Ecological signs (triggers): Openness to individuals, spots, and things related to earlier medication utilizing encounters that might cause quick and overpowering desire;

• Stress: Dependent people encountering pressure as a hankering;

• Psychological instability;

• Drug withdrawal: Side effects of both psychological instability and withdrawal lead to hankering to assume clients partner use with alleviation of these side effects.

The CIM Model consolidates four help conveyance components:

• Backslide Anticipation Studio,

• Individual guiding,

• Clinical/mental administration,

• Evaluating for progressing drug use.

Issues in mental administration of hankering

People with a molding history of over and over encountering the powerful psychopharmacologic impacts of medications and liquor on cognizance have discovered that psychoactive substances are solid, fast, and viable means by which mental uneasiness can be felt better [5]. The more noteworthy the uneasiness, the more prominent the longing to get away from inconvenience, and subsequently more grounded the desire. Hence, the aversive mental encounters can be seen as a rebuffing occasion, the expulsion or weakening of which is capable of adversely supporting. Because of the constant person of long haul substance use, experienced substance clients may not be in every case profoundly mindful of the exact idea of the mental encounters that they might be consequently self-regulating and subsequently moderately ignorant about the mental premise of their desire.

This likewise might be the aftereffect of ongoing alteration of mental occasions with psychoactive substances by which medications and liquor are capably used to try not to completely encounter mental occasions in any event, when expected to be horrendous or poisonous. In this situation, the substance is utilized not exclusively to get away from aversive cognizant encounters yet, in addition, to stay away from them. Therefore, straightforwardly asking a substance client for what good reason the person desires liquor or medications might be inefficient. By rethinking the hankering explanation, attributes of the mental experience (i.e., considerations, sentiments, sensations, recollections, and pictures) changed by substance use can be made expressed. Such data can explain the mental premise of medication impacts, drug inclinations, and medication anticipations and feature lacks in nonpharmacological adapting abilities and mental self-regulation.

There is a need to create some distance from clinically based and shortsighted pharmacological administration of hankering and move towards an all-encompassing group approach. Propels in comprehension of the idea of hankering are permitting further advancement of promising new medicines. With the appearance of new, encouraging administration techniques pointed toward forestalling backslide, there is a more noteworthy expectation for better and supported administration of hankering substance use jumble. Bringing about better adherence to treatment, lesser backslide, and cost trouble for patients. There is additionally a need for more exploration with a huge populace test on the lines of mental administration to demonstrate its viability.

Chapter 2

The motivations behind why smoking is awful for you

Smoking and wellbeing

Mind

Cardiovascular framework

Bones

Resistant framework

Lungs

Mouth

Propagation

Skin

Disease

Advantages of stopping

Smoking harms practically every organ in the body. Individuals can essentially lessen their possibility of smoking-related infection by surrendering it.

Smoking is the main preventable reason for early illness and demise in the US. Quitting any pretense of smoking is hard for some individuals, yet the quantity of previous smokers is expanding constantly.

As per the Communities for Infectious prevention and Anticipation (CDC)Trusted Source, current smoking in the U.S. has declined from 20.9% in 2005 to 13.7% in 2018. The quantity of smokers who have stopped is additionally rising.

In this article, we take a gander at the well-being effect of smoking, remembering its belongings for the cerebrum, heart, lungs, and safe framework. We additionally examine the advantages of stopping.

How does smoking influence well-being?
Consistently, over 480,000 people trusted Source bite the dust in the U.S. because of tobacco-related illnesses — around 1 of every 5 of all passings — as per the American Malignant Growth Society.

engine vehicle wounds

liquor or unlawful medication use
gun-related episodes
Tobacco contains noxious substances that influence individuals' well-being. Two of these toxic substances are:

Carbon monoxide. Vehicle exhaust vapor likewise produces this substance, and it is lethal in huge portions. It replaces oxygen in the blood and keeps the organs from oxygen, preventing them from working accurately.
Tar. This is a tacky, earthy-colored substance that covers the lungs and influences relaxation.
While the measurements are disturbing, it is critical to remember that quitting any pretense of smoking lessens the gamble of sickness emphatically.

Underneath, we talk about the effect smoking can have on various pieces of the body.

Cerebrum

Smoking can improve the probability of having a stroke by 2-4 timesTrusted Source. Strokes can cause cerebrum harm and passing.

One way that stroke can cause cerebrum injury is through a mind aneurysm, which happens when the mass of a vein debilitates and makes a lump. This lump can explode and cause a subarachnoid drain, which can prompt a stroke.

Heart

Synthetic compounds in tobacco smoke increment the opportunity for heart issues and cardiovascular illnesses.

Smoking causes atherosclerosis, which is when plaque develops in the blood and adheres to the supply route walls. This makes them smaller, diminishing the bloodstream and expanding the gamble of blood clusters.

Smoking additionally harms the veins, making them thicker and smaller. This makes it harder for blood to stream and increments circulatory strain and pulse.

Smoking has joined with the accompanying cardiovascular circumstances:

coronary illness, one of the main sources of death trusted Source in the U.S
a respiratory failure, as smoking copies the gamble of a coronary episode
blockages that decrease the bloodstream to the skin and legs
stroke because of blood clumps or burst veins in the cerebrum
Indeed, even smokers who smoke 5 or fewer trusted Source cigarettes daily might foster early indications of cardiovascular sickness.

Carbon monoxide and nicotine make the heart work harder and quicker. This implies that smoking makes it more testing to work out. An absence of activity further expands the gamble of medical issues.

Bones

As per the Public Foundation for Wellbeing (NIH), smoking decreases bone thickness, making the bones more vulnerable and weak. Smoking can likewise disable bone mending after a crack.

Scientists find it challenging to say whether this is an immediate impact of smoking, or because of other gamble factors predominant in individuals who smoke. These incorporate lower body weight and doing less actual activity.

This might influence females more trusted Sources than guys. Females are more inclined to osteoporosis and broken bones.

Stopping smoking, considerably further down the road, can assist with restricting bone misfortune connected with smoking.

.

Resistant framework

The resistant framework safeguards the body against contamination and illness.

Crohn's infection

rheumatoid joint pain

ulcerative colitis

fundamental lupus erythematosus

Smoking additionally joins with type 2 diabetes.

Lungs

The lungs are maybe the clearest organ that smoking affects.

It frequently requires numerous years before an individual notification any side effects of smoking-related lung illness. This implies that individuals may not get a conclusion until the sickness is very best in class.

Smoking can affect the lungs in more ways than one. The essential reason trusted Source is that smoking harms the aviation routes and air sacs — known as alveoli — in the lungs.

Mouth

Smoking can severely affect oral well-being and may cause:

halitosis, or awful breath
stained teeth
dry mouth
the diminished feeling of taste

Smoking bothers the gum tissues. The American Dental Affiliation (ADA) expresses that smoking expands the gamble of gum illness, which can add to halitosis.

Proliferation

Smoking could also trusted Source at any point to influence the regenerative framework and richness.

Females who smoke can have more trouble becoming pregnant. In guys, smoking can cause barrenness by harming veins in the penis. It can likewise harm sperm and influence, sperm count.

As per a few examinations, guys who smoke have a lower sperm count Confided in Sourcethan the people who don't.

Smoking while pregnant expands various dangers for the child, including:

untimely birth
pregnancy misfortune
low birth weight
abrupt newborn child passing disorder
newborn child ailments

Skin
Smoking lessens how much oxygen that can arrive at the skin. These velocities up the

maturing system and can cause the skin to seem dull or dark.

Smoking can cause:

facial kinks, particularly around the lips
loose eyelids
lopsided skin shading, like a yellow or dim tone
dry, coarse skin
transitory yellowing of the fingers and fingernails
Smoking diminishes how rapidly skin wounds recuperate, expands the gamble of skin diseases, and builds the seriousness of skin conditions, including psoriasis.

Smoking and malignant growth risk
Smoking builds the gamble of many sorts of malignant growth. As indicated by the Public Disease InstituteTrusted Source, tobacco smoke contains around 7,000 synthetic substances, of which no less than 69 can cause malignant growth.

Figures from the American Malignant growth SocietyTrusted Source express that smoking causes around 30% of all disease passings in the U.S. and 80% of all cellular breakdown in the lungs passings.

Cellular breakdown in the lungs is the main source of disease passing in all kinds of people. It is one of the hardest to treat.

Smoking is a gamble factor for the accompanying malignant growths:

mouth
larynx, or voice box
pharynx, or throat
throat, the cylinder associating the mouth and stomach
kidney
cervix
liver
bladder
pancreas

stomach
colon
myeloid leukemia
Stogies, pipe-smoking, menthol cigarettes, biting tobacco, and different types of tobacco all cause malignant growth and other medical issues. There is no protected method for utilizing tobacco.

Peruse more about how smoking influences the body here.

The advantages of stopping
While the measurements are disturbing, fortunately stopping smoking decreases the gamble of sickness and passing fundamentally. The dangers drop further, the more extended an individual ceases smoking.

Some examination says that stopping before the age of 40 lessens the gamble of biting the dust from smoking-related illness by around 90%.

These statisticsTrusted Sources show the medical advantages of stopping smoking:

Cardiovascular dangers: Following 1 year of stopping, the gamble of having a coronary failure drops strongly.
Stroke: Within 2-5 years, the gamble of a stroke lessens to a portion of that of a non-smoker.
Tumors: The dangers for mouth, throat, throat, and bladder disease drop by half in no less than 5 years of stopping, and 10 years for the cellular breakdown in the lungs.
Not long after stopping, individuals experience the accompanying medical advantages that can fundamentally work on their satisfaction and act as tokens of the medical advantages that stopping can have:

breathing becomes more straightforward
day to day hacking and wheezing decrease then vanishes

the feeling of taste and smell improve
exercise and exercises become more straightforward
flow to the hands and feet moves along
Peruse more about what happens when you quit smoking here.

However stopping can be unpleasant, individuals frequently begin to see their everyday feelings of anxiety are a lot lower than when they were smoking for a half year or something like that.

Stopping smoking is an alternate excursion for everybody, and what works for one individual won't necessarily in all cases work for the following. Evaluate perhaps one or two methods for seeing which ones work best.

While attempting to stop smoking, these tips might help:

Make arrangements of motivations behind why it is smart to stop. Peruse these when the compulsion to smoke strikes.

Utilize an application to keep tabs on your development. Arriving at achievements, like a day without smoking, can assist with spurring an individual to proceed. There are many free and paid applications available.

Attempt nicotine substitution items. Nicotine patches, gums, and capsules can assist with diminishing desires, making it simpler to oppose at a specific second.

Many individuals find that connecting with a medical services supplier for help can assist them with stopping for good. A specialist can endorse a drug, for example, varenicline (Chantix).

Smoking can influence sexual well-being in all kinds of people. Young ladies who smoke and are on chemical-based contraception techniques like the Pill, the fix, or the ring have a higher gamble of serious medical conditions, similar to respiratory failures.

Furthermore, getting pregnant, and smoking can make that harder.

Other than these drawn-out issues, the synthetic substances in cigarettes and different items additionally can influence the body rapidly. Adolescent smokers can have a large number of these issues:

Terrible breath. Cigarettes leave smokers with a condition called halitosis or enduring terrible breath.
Terrible smelling garments and hair. The smell of old smoke will in general keep going — on individuals' clothing, yet on their hair, furniture, and vehicles. It's difficult to get the smell of smoke out.
Inconvenience keeping up in sports. Smokers as a rule can't contend well with nonsmokers. Actual impacts of smoking, similar to a quick heartbeat, diminished dissemination, and windedness, hurt sports execution.

The more serious gamble of injury and more slow mending time. Smoking damages the body's capacity to make collagen. So normal game wounds, for example, harm to ligaments and tendons, will recuperate more leisurely in smokers than nonsmokers.

Expanded hazard of sickness. Concentrates show that smokers become ill more with colds, influenza, bronchitis, and pneumonia than nonsmokers. Furthermore, individuals with some ailments, similar to asthma, get more debilitated if they smoke (and frequently if they're simply around individuals who smoke). Teenagers who smoke as a method for dealing with their weight frequently light up as opposed to eating. So their bodies can come up short on supplements expected to develop, create, and ward off sickness well

Chapter 3

What's in store when you quit smoking

Stopping smoking is perhaps the best thing you will at any point accomplish for your well-being.

Withdrawal can be testing, however, it can help to assume you view the side effects as signs that your body is recuperating.

Normal side effects include desires, fretfulness, inconvenience thinking or dozing, crabbiness, nervousness, expansions in craving, and weight gain.

Many individuals find withdrawal side effects vanish following two to about a month.

Quitline is accessible to assist you with stopping, 8 am - 8 pm, Monday to Friday.

Changing your routine can assist with staying away from those triggers that tell your cerebrum it's the ideal opportunity for a smoke.

Quit smoking drugs can assist you with stopping smoking.

On this page

Side effects when you quit smoking

Feeling close to home when you quit

Weight gain and stopping smoking

Overseeing smoking withdrawal side effects

Overseeing pressure when you quit smoking

Expenses of smoking

Advantages of stopping smoking

If you begin smoking once more

Help is accessible to stop

Where to find support

At the point when you choose to stop smoking, it can assist with figuring out what's in store as you work through the cycle. Certain individuals have a couple of gentle side effects when they quit however others think that it is more enthusiastically.

While withdrawal can be testing, it can help on the off chance that you view the side effects as signs that your body is recuperating from the harm smoking has caused.

Many individuals find withdrawal side effects vanish following two to about a month, even though for certain individuals they might endure longer. Side effects will quite often travel every which way throughout that time. Keep in mind, it will pass, and you will feel improved on the off chance that you hold tight and quit forever.

Side effects when you quit smoking
Normal side effects you might insight during your recuperation include:

desires - these might be areas of strength for being first, yet they normally just last a couple of moments. Assuming you oppose everyone they will get less strong in time
fretfulness and inconvenience thinking or resting - these will pass as your body becomes acclimated to not smoking.

Unwinding and profound breathing can help.
peevishness, outrage, tension, discouraged state of mind - this is all typical: don't overreact. Simply acknowledge that you will be close to home for some time and that it will pass
expansion in craving and weight gain - this might most recent a little while. Preparing can help. Better Wellbeing Channel has tips on overseeing weight gain when you quit.
More uncommon side effects you might insight - which will likewise pass - include:

cold side effects like hacking and wheezing
blockage
discombobulation or wooziness
mouth ulcers.
Over the long haul, you will find these side effects become more fragile, and you will contemplate smoking less. If you have extreme or durable side effects, it could assist with examining them with well-being proficiency or a Quitline guide. It could

likewise assist with utilizing nicotine substitution treatment or endorsed quit-smoking tablets. For additional tips go to Hankering a Cigarette at present.

Caffeine (for instance, in espresso, chocolate, and cola sodas) and liquor are likewise impacted by tobacco smoke. Eliminating beverages or food sources with caffeine when you quit smoking is suggested. It's critical to talk with your PCP about halting smoking assuming you drink liquor.

Feeling profound when you quit

In the primary long periods when you quit smoking, the close-to-home high points and low points could feel like a rollercoaster ride. Rolling out huge improvements in your day-to-day existence can normally prompt uplifted feelings.

Certain individuals portray quitting any pretense of smoking as feeling like you're losing a companion. However long you comprehend that this is only a phase and what you're feeling is typical, you can ride through the difficult situations and subside into feeling more certain without cigarettes.

Knowing how rapidly you will recuperate by stopping can help:

In no less than six hours your pulse will slow and your circulatory strain will turn out to be more steady.
In something like one day your circulatory system will be nearly nicotine free, the degree of carbon monoxide in your blood will have dropped, and oxygen will arrive at your heart and muscles all the more without any problem.
In no less than a multi-week, your feeling of taste and smell might have gotten to the next level.
In somewhere around 90 days you will hack and wheeze less, your safe capability and flow to your hands and feet will be

improving, and your lungs will get better at eliminating bodily fluid, tar, and residue.

In a half year, your feelings of anxiety are probably going to have dropped, and you are less inclined to hack up mucus.

Following one year your lungs will be better and breathing will be more straightforward than if you'd continued to smoke.

Within two to five years your gamble of coronary illness will have dropped essentially (and will keep on doing as such after some time).

In no less than five years, a lady's gamble of cervical malignant growth will be equivalent to on the off chance that she had never smoked.

Following 10 to 15 years your gamble of cellular breakdown in the lungs will be a portion of that of a person of a comparative age who continues to smoke.

Following 20 years your gamble of cardiovascular failure and stroke will be like that of somebody who has never smoked.

Weight gain and stopping smoking

Weight gain isn't in every case part of stopping smoking yet it is normal. You might find you feel hungrier than normal after you quit - this is a typical withdrawal side effect and it will settle down with time. It can assist with preparing and having a lot of solid snacks in the kitchen, like nuts and natural products, and disposing of unhealthy food from your home.

Assuming you in all actuality do put on weight in the good 'old days, do whatever it takes not to be too severe with yourself. By stopping smoking you're doing extraordinary things for your well-being.

Overseeing smoking withdrawal side effects
Even though withdrawal side effects can feel testing, there are ways you can assist yourself with remaining inspired:

Keep a rundown of reasons you have chosen to stop and save it convenient for those minutes when you're enticed to smoke.

Make arrangements and remain occupied.
Connect with loved ones to assist with diverting you from your desires and keep you spurred.
Recall the four Ds:
defer following up on the desire for five minutes and it will generally pass
do some profound relaxing
hydrate, or
accomplish something different.
Schedules to assist you with overseeing desires
Perhaps the greatest test many individuals face at the beginning of stopping is normal desires. A few desires are your body truly needing nicotine, however, some are likewise connected with your day-to-day schedules.

Changing your routine can assist with keeping away from those triggers that tell your cerebrum it's the ideal opportunity for a smoke.

Here are a few thoughts for exercises to do as opposed to smoking at those times you as a rule go after the cigarettes:

at the crack of dawn - have a shower
with espresso or tea - change to an alternate beverage, an alternate cup, or change where you drink it
at morning tea - sit in a better place or with various individuals, read a magazine, or take a look at your virtual entertainment
at the PC at home - move your work area or refurbish to change the look
after a feast - take a walk
after work - practice or reflect
before supper - make your supper time prior
with liquor - change to an alternate kind of drink or hold your beverage in your smoking hand
as you plan your next task - inhale profoundly
as a prize - pay attention to music or have a piece natural product

at the point when you're with an individual who's smoking - bite gum or bring a water bottle

before the TV - move the furniture around, hold a pressure ball, and do some simple stretches

before bed - have a warm beverage or perused a book.

Keep in mind, each time you oppose that desire and accomplish something different rather it's a triumph in your mission to stop: you're assisting your cerebrum with breaking that connection between the action and the cigarette.

The more choices you need to divert yourself, the better. The following are a couple of additional thoughts you can attempt whenever:

Taste a glass of water gradually.

Play with a pet.

Call a companion.

Play a game on your telephone.

Ask your accomplice or a companion for a shoulder rub.
Attempt some cultivating.
Put on some hand cream.
Do a jigsaw puzzle or crossword.
Strip an orange.
Contemplate the reasons you're stopping and imagine a positive future.
Overseeing pressure when you quit smoking
It will require investment to sink into new schedules and track down better approaches to manage pressure now that smoking isn't a choice.

The pressure discharge you feel when you have a cigarette is short-lived. It doesn't take care of your concerns, it just moves your concentration and feeds the smoking pressure cycle.

Research lets us know that individuals who smoke will quite often have higher feelings of anxiety than non-smokers. A great many people find that their feelings of anxiety are lower a half year in the wake of stopping than they were before they stopped.

Perhaps the greatest test you'll confront when you quit is tracking down a better approach to take 'personal time - at work, when you initially return home, after supper, and at different times when you simply need some break.

You could find it supportive to make an exceptional space for yourself to unwind. Or on the other hand, you could have a go at returning to an old side interest or beginning another one.

Perceive How to manage pressure when you quit for thoughts on incredible break exercises.

Expenses of smoking
There is no reason for harping on how much cash you have proactively spent on smoking. In any case, you may as yet set aside cash if

you quit, and the sooner you quit, the more cash you will save.

On the off chance that you smoke a bunch of 20 cigarettes per day at $27, you will save around $10,000 every year. Contemplating how else you might want to manage that cash can be an extraordinary inspiration to adhere to your quit plan.

Attempt this cost mini-computer to perceive the amount you can save by quitting any pretense of smoking.

Advantages of stopping smoking
Stopping is perhaps the best thing you will at any point accomplish for your well-being. It can influence your life in manners you may not envision.

Advantages to your well-being and life from stopping smoking include:

Your feeling of taste and smell might improve, so you might partake in your food more.

Practicing to expand your wellness will become simpler.

You will be liberated from the problems of smoking, like resembling smoke, or continuously ensuring you have an adequate number of cigarettes.

Your ripeness levels will improve (in all kinds of people), and if you're a lady, your possibilities of having a solid pregnancy and child will likewise increment.

You will save a large number of dollars a year that you can save or spend on different things.

Your loved ones will likewise benefit because:

You won't jeopardize their well-being with recycled smoke any longer

Your kids will be less in danger from bronchitis, pneumonia, asthma, meningitis, and ear contamination.

Assuming you begin smoking once more

On the off chance that you have a cigarette, don't blame it to return to smoking.

Eliminate yourself from the circumstance. Take a walk, take a full breath or have a beverage of water, and inquire as to whether you truly need to smoke once more. Do whatever it takes not to squander your energy on self-fault. All things being equal, treat that cigarette as a sign to modify your stopping technique.

Assuming you've attempted a few times to quit any pretense of smoking and you haven't succeeded at this point, don't lose trust. It's normal for individuals to attempt to stop various times before they quit smoking for good.

Next time you quit, invest some energy pondering what has worked for you previously, and what moves made you return to smoking. Then make arrangements for how you will respond this time when those enticements come up once more.

Help is accessible to stop

To figure out the entirety of your choices, converse with your PCP or drug specialist about how they can assist you with stopping, and call Quitline. Quitline is a free phone support administration. Quitline guides are prepared to listen cautiously and give you support fit to your requirements. You don't need to do this by yourself. Furthermore, self-control isn't the main instrument available to you - you can purchase nicotine patches, capsules, or gum and endorsed quit-smoking tablets all the more efficiently with content from your PCP.

Your primary care physician or drug specialist can prompt you on which quit-smoking prescription would suit you and how your standard meds might require changing when you stop smoking. You can likewise go online at quit.org.au and make your quit plan with simple-to-find data fit to you.

You can pursue Quit Mail. North of 12 weeks Quit Mail will send you customary messages following your well-being and cash gains, in addition to heaps of tips to assist you with remaining quit.

Before you quit, it's wise to have an arrangement for getting past these withdrawals. You'll make some simpler memories assuming you're intellectually ready and have a few methodologies for how to think about your side effects.

Know What's in store

Anybody who's stopped (or attempted to stop) smoking will let you know that the main seven-day stretch of withdrawal is horrible. In the 3 to 4 days that your body is cleaning out the nicotine off of that last cigarette, you will feel genuinely awful - -

and your psychological state and feelings will be all around the guide.

In any case, it will get better after that. You'll improve truly, and your psychological side effects will likewise begin to disappear throughout the following couple of weeks.

You probably won't have these side effects, and you could observe that some are more straightforward to deal with than others. In any case, you ought to know about them so they don't shock you.

A few side effects, for example, migraines and hacks, you'll simply need to get past. In any case, you can play a functioning job in guaranteeing that you endure the others.

Step-by-step instructions to Manage Desires
Desires are the longest-enduring and most grounded withdrawal side effect. They can begin in something like 30 minutes of your

last cigarette, as the nicotine begins to wear off and your body needs more.

The most horrendously terrible of the actual desires will be over in a couple of days when all the nicotine has left your framework. However at that point come the psychological desires, which can keep going for half a month.

Approach it slowly and carefully. Make an effort not to stress over how you'll traverse the following couple of weeks. Each need should endure simply 15 to 20 minutes. There are a ton of ways of outliving a desire, so it pays to keep a psychological rundown of things you can do, such as:

Keep your mouth occupied with gum, hard treats, and crunchy (good) food
Use nicotine substitution treatment, similar to gum, tablets, or the fix
Take a walk or do a few fast activities while a hankering hits

Make a beeline for a public spot where you can't smoke
Call or text a companion
Take full breaths
Begin another everyday practice for times when you normally smoke
Keep away from triggers that make you need to smoke, similar as liquor, caffeine, or individuals you realize who smoke
Recollect why you quit

Taking care of Other Withdrawal Side effects
Nicotine substitution treatment, besides assisting with desires, can likewise ease different side effects by giving a little hit of nicotine without the other risky synthetic compounds tracked down in cigarettes.

Biting nicotine gum or sucking on a tablet could help when you're worried or feeling restless.

It assists with remaining occupied while you're attempting to overcome hankering. However, dialing back is likewise really smart. Attempt yoga, contemplation, and profound breathing when withdrawal begins to get to you.

Cigarettes contain synthetics that check your hunger, so food desires are likewise a major piece of withdrawal. Acquiring 5 to 10 pounds in the initial not many weeks is normal. Eating can likewise turn into a movement that assists you with managing nicotine desires. Be aware of this and keep sound tidbits available.

Most importantly, remain fixed on the 10,000-foot view and recollect that withdrawal will before long be previously.

Chapter 4

It is widely accepted that the nicotine in cigarettes is highly addictive, but people struggling with mental health issues often turn to cigarettes for reasons that go beyond their addictive qualities. For instance, many people smoke as a coping mechanism to deal with difficult feelings. In addition, despite their negative health effects, cigarettes are still largely viewed by society as an "acceptable" addiction in comparison with other substances.

The reality? "[Smoking] is a devastating addiction and a difficult one to quit," says Gary Tedeschi, clinical director of the California Smokers' Helpline and a member of the American Counseling Association. "This clientele [those with mental illness], in particular, need the encouragement and support to go forward [with quitting], and many of them want to, despite what people might think. ... To let people continue to smoke because 'it's not as bad [as other addictions] is missing a really important chance to help someone get healthier."

To drive home his point, Tedeschi points to a statistic from the 2014 release of The Health Consequences of Smoking — 50 Years of Progress: A Report of the Surgeon General, which says that more than 480,000 people die annually in the United States from causes related to cigarette smoking. Close to half of the Americans who die from tobacco-related causes are people with mental illness or substance abuse disorders, Tedeschi says.

In Tedeschi's view, the statistics connecting smoking to mental illness are "so obvious that it's almost an ethical and moral responsibility to help this population quit."

Tobacco use "is always part of a package" that clients will bring to counseling, Brooks says. In his experience as an addictions counselor, smoking is often piled on top of a laundry list of other challenges that may include alcohol or drug addiction, depression, a marriage that is on the rocks, the loss of a job, or financial trouble.

"They're on the train to destruction, and their nicotine use, in their minds, is on the back end [in terms of importance]. ... Is smoking related to what their presenting issue is? Chances are it probably connects somehow. Don't be afraid to bring it up," advises Brooks, co-author of the book A Contemporary Approach to Substance Use Disorders and Addiction Counseling, which is published by ACA.

Tedeschi, a nationally certified counselor, and licensed psychologist note that many people who call the California Smokers'

Helpline are struggling with comorbid conditions or mental illness in addition to tobacco use. The phone line is one in a system of "quitlines" operating in each of the 50 U.S. states, the District of Columbia, Puerto Rico, and Guam.

For clients struggling with mental health issues, smoking may serve as a coping mechanism to deal with uncomfortable feelings or anxiety, Brooks says. Years ago, when smoking was still allowed in many indoor spaces, Brooks led group counseling in detox, outpatient, and inpatient addiction facilities. "When powerful emotions would come up in the group, [clients] would fire up cigarette after cigarette to deal with those feelings and quell anxiety," he recalls.

With this in mind, counselors should help prepare clients for the irritability, anxiety, and other uncomfortable feelings they are likely to experience when they attempt to stop smoking cigarettes. "Talk about what it will feel like to be anxious and not smoke" and how they plan to handle those feelings, Brooks says. "... If a person has anxiety or depression and stops smoking, what initially happens is they could get more depressed or more anxious without nicotine to quell the emotion."

The counselors interviewed for this article urge practitioners to ask every single client about their tobacco use during the intake process, no matter what the person's presenting problem is. "If you're helping them to get mentally and physically healthier, this [quitting smoking] is a very critical part of the overall wellness picture," Tedeschi says.

Counselors shouldn't be afraid to ask their clients whether they smoke, says Greg Harms, a licensed clinical professional counselor (LCPC), certified addictions specialist, and alcohol and drug counselor with a private practice in Chicago. "It can feel weird the first couple of times, especially if this is not your area of expertise," says Harms, who does postdoctoral work at Diamond Headache Clinic in Chicago, an inpatient unit for people with chronic headaches. "A lot of times, clients have heard all the bad stuff about smoking. A lot of them, deep down, know they'd be better off if they were to quit smoking. They may have failed so many times in the past that they're discouraged. They might be hesitant to bring it up because this is a counselor and not the [medical] doctor. If you bring it up, more often than not, the client is going to engage with that. Even if they don't, if it's not the right time for them, you've planted that seed. ... It might come to fruition down the road. I'd much rather plant that seed than not say anything at all."

When Harms was a counseling graduate student, he completed an internship at the Anixter Center, a Chicago agency that serves clients with disabilities. While there, he worked as part of a grant-funded program for smoking cessation for people with disabilities that was spearheaded by the American Lung Association.

If a client doesn't feel ready to begin the quitting process right away, the counselor can put the topic on the back burner to address again once the client has made progress on other presenting problems or has forged a stronger relationship with the practitioner. However, that shouldn't mean that the topic is off the table completely, Harms says. A counselor should talk regularly with the client about quitting smoking, even if it's only for a few minutes each session.

"Give them a little nugget of information [about quitting], and then you can focus on what they're there for," Harms says. "Help them find ways to deal with their presenting problem, then they'll trust you. Once they're in a better place, revisit [the idea of quitting]. We don't have to address it and get their buy-in during the first session. It would be fantastic if that were the case, but it's OK if it's not. In most cases, time is on our side to develop the relationship, plant the seed and revisit it. If the client is not ready, we can harp on [quitting] all we want, [but] it won't do anything."

"You have to take the client's lead and go at the pace they're willing," Harms continues. "Don't push. Respect their decision. Even if they're not ready for [quitting], let them know that [you're] there for them and respect their autonomy to make that decision."

Positioned to help

Counselors are particularly suited to help clients quit smoking because the profession has an array of tools focused on behavior modification, Tedeschi asserts. Motivational interviewing, cognitive behavior therapy, acceptance and commitment therapy, and other models can be useful in helping clients stop smoking. But techniques from any therapy model that counselors are comfortable using can be adapted to help clients navigate the challenge of quitting, Tedeschi says, especially when combined appropriately with pharmacologic aids approved by the Food and Drug Administration.

"We're in the business of helping people change. The principles that a counselor uses to help someone understand an issue and begin to take steps toward change apply to smoking cessation as well," Tedeschi says. "Counselors help people understand their motivation to change and help them come up with a plan to change."

Harms agrees, noting that in most cases, a counselor will have significantly more time with a client than a medical professional will. Instead of “hitting [the client] over the head” with the dangers of smoking, Harms says, a counselor can afford to focus on the positive, use a strengths-based approach and build on what the client wants to work toward rather than what he or she wants to avoid.

“We [counselors] are so strengths-based. It’s our natural inclination to tell the client, ‘Yes, you’re strong enough to do this,’ rather than [taking] a scare approach,” Harms says. “We can find their strength and have that unconditional positive regard for them, regardless of how long it’s taking. We have the patience to sit with a client as they’re going through [quitting]. We can build that relationship and be a resource.”

Start small

Tedeschi recommends that counselors use the “five A’s” to discuss smoking with clients. In this approach, a practitioner should:

Ask each client about his or her tobacco use
Advise all tobacco users to quit
Assess whether the client is ready to quit
Assist the client with a quit plan
Arrange follow-up contact to mitigate relapse
Each of these steps is important, but providing support and follow-up as the client begins to quit is particularly critical, Tedeschi says.

"The first week of quitting is the hardest. If [a counselor] waits for a week to talk to the client, you could lose about 60 percent of people back to relapse," he says. "If someone can quit for two weeks, their risk of relapse drops dramatically."

If clients resist the idea of quitting or do not feel ready to quit entirely, Tedeschi suggests that counselors work with them to stop smoking for one day or even just an afternoon. During this time, have clients monitor how they felt: How was their anxiety level? What were their cravings like? This technique can introduce the idea of stopping and preparing clients for the quitting process, he says.

Brooks recommends using motivational interviewing to help clients make the life change to quit smoking. “Nicotine is a drug, and it’s no different than if [clients] were to say they want to stop drinking. Work with their motivation to identify what they can do for that,” he says.

Part of the quitting process involves clients going through an identity shift, Tedeschi notes. Clients can be behaving as nonsmokers – abstaining from cigarettes – long before they make the mental leap that they are no longer smokers, he says. It is important for clients to make that mental shift from “a smoker who is not smoking” to a “nonsmoker,” Tedeschi says. Counselors need to work with these clients to identify as and accept the nonsmoker label. “As long as someone calls [himself or herself] a smoker, they will be open to turning back to cigarettes,” he explains.

Kicking the habit

Counselors can use the following tips and techniques to better equip clients to meet the challenge to stop smoking.

Set a quit date. This is an important step, but one that clients must take the lead on and choose for themselves, Tedeschi says. Research shows that simply cutting back without setting a quit date isn’t very effective, he adds. The behavioral patterns that often accompany smoking (for example, smoking after eating or taking smoke breaks at work) make it very hard to keep tobacco use at a low level. Setting a quit date creates accountability and is a “sign of seriousness,” he says. At the same time, be flexible. "For some people, it's just too hard to think about [sticking to a quit date]," Tedeschi says. "For some – especially those who are struggling with other substances – they need to take one day at a time."

Be aware of psychotropic medications. Counselors should be aware that if clients are taking prescription medicines for anxiety, depression, bipolar disorder, or other mental illnesses, their dosages might need to be adjusted as they quit smoking. Nicotine is a stimulant, so it speeds up a person's metabolism. This means a person who smokes will burn through psychotropic medications faster than someone who doesn't smoke, Harms explains. Counselors should be certain to talk this through with clients and work with their doctors to modify their dosages, he says. "This is especially noticeable with mood stabilizers. It's acute with bipolar disorder," Harms says.

The same holds with caffeine, Tedeschi notes. After they quit smoking, clients may notice that they get jittery from caffeine and may need to cut back on their coffee intake.

Use cognitive strategies. Counselors can help clients create a list of personal reasons why they want to stop smoking — beyond the health implications, Tedeschi says. The list doesn't need to be long, but the reasons need to be compelling and motivating enough to carry clients through a nicotine craving. For example, one of Tedeschi's clients wanted to quit because his young grandson asked him to. As a reminder, the client kept a toy car that belonged to his grandson in his pocket. "When he had a craving [for a cigarette], he would pull [the toy car] out of his pocket, look at it, hold it and squeeze it," Tedeschi says. "It helped."

Turn over a new leaf. As they quit smoking, encourage clients to organize, clean, and purge their homes and cars of smoking-related materials such as ashtrays, advises ACA member Pari Sharif, an LPC with a practice in Franklin Lakes, New Jersey. That action will help clients turn a new page mentally and start fresh, she says. Sharif also encourages clients to air out their homes and clean their closets so their clothes and furniture no longer smell like smoke.

On a similar note, if clients have a certain mug that they always use to drink coffee while smoking, Harms suggests that they get a new mug. Or if they always stopped at a certain gas station to buy cigarettes, he suggests that they now change where they buy gas.

When cravings strike, breathe. Sharif, a certified tobacco treatment specialist, introduces breathing techniques to all of her smoking cessation clients. She asks these clients to take measured breaths for roughly two minutes, inhaling while slowly counting to four, then exhaling for four counts.

"Instead of the reflex habit to grab a cigarette, take a moment to stop and ask why. Be more in control of yourself and your mind," she tells clients. "Pause to do breathing and body scanning from head to toe. Ask yourself, 'What am I doing? Why do I need this [cigarette] to calm down?' ... [Through breathing exercises,] your breath becomes deeper and deeper. Close your eyes. Your body starts relaxing and your anxiety level goes down."

Sharif also recommends that clients download a meditation app for their smartphones and use a journal to record how they're feeling when cigarette cravings strike. This helps them log and identify which situations and emotions are triggering their need for nicotine,
she explains.

Get to the root of it. Asking clients about the circumstances that first caused them to start smoking can help in identifying what triggers their nicotine use and the bigger issues that may need to be addressed through counseling, Sharif says. In some cases, a specific traumatic event or stressor caused the person to start smoking. In other instances, it was a learned behavior because everyone in the household smoked as the client was growing up. “Find out when they started smoking and why,” Sharif says. “Gradually, when they become more aware of themselves, they quit.”

Change social patterns. Cigarettes are often used as a coping mechanism when people experience anxiety in social situations, Harms says, so clients may need to focus on social skills as they start the process of quitting smoking.

“[Cigarettes] are their way to socialize and get out and meet people. If you have social anxiety, you can still go up to someone and ask for a cigarette or ask for a light. It's programmed socialization," Harms explains. "It gives you an excuse to be close to people, and feel more sociable. If you take away their cigarettes, you've got to replace that."

Brooks agrees, noting that clients who smoke likely have friends who are also smokers. For example, he says, it is not uncommon to see people smoking and talking together outside of Alcoholics Anonymous meetings. Counselors can help clients prepare to avoid situations where smoking is expected and practice asking people not to smoke around them, Brooks says. Counselors can also support clients in creating social networks of people who don't smoke, including support groups for ex-smokers, he adds.

Break behavioral habits. Similarly, Brooks says, counselors can help clients change the behavioral habits they connect to smoking, such as starting the morning by reading the paper, drinking coffee, and smoking a cigarette. Counselors can suggest activities and new rituals replace the old ones, such as taking a daily walk, he says.

Harms encourages clients to replace their former smoke breaks with "clean air breaks." They can still take their normal time outside, but instead of smoking, he suggests that they walk around the block, sit and read a book, eat an apple or use their smartphones outdoors. If they had a favorite smoking spot outside, he urges them to find a new place to go instead.

Find comforting substitutes. "The whole ritual of lighting up a cigarette — tapping the pack to pull out a cigarette and flicking the lighter — the behaviors that go with [smoking] can be very comforting," Harms says. "Sometimes that's what's so hard to break — the behaviors that go with it."

Tedeschi recommends that counselors work with clients to have comforting alternatives ready to go even before the clients attempt to quit smoking. It is hard for people to figure out alternatives in the heat of the moment when a craving strikes, he explains. Tedeschi offers several possible substitutes for consideration: sugar-free gum, beef jerky, cinnamon sticks, and even drinking straws cut into cigarette-sized lengths through which clients can inhale and exhale.

If clients are comforted by having something in their hands, Brooks suggests keeping a pen, stress ball, or prayer beads nearby. Staying hydrated and carrying a water bottle can also help these clients, Tedeschi adds. Most of all, counselors should work toward the idea of replenishment and filling in where clients feel they are losing something, he says.

Don't dismiss pharmacotherapy. A wide variety of quitting aids are available, from nicotine patches, lozenges, and gum, to prescription pills such as Chantix. The counselors interviewed for this article agree that these stop-smoking aids can be helpful when used alongside counseling. However, Tedeschi says, counselors should work with their clients' physicians when such medications are being used, or make sure that clients are talking with their physicians. Counselors should also be aware of the potential side effects that these medications can have, such as aggressive behavior.

Chapter 5

After Quit Day

Have a severe 'no puff' strategy

Focus on not having even a solitary puff after you have stopped. Having 'only one cigarette' quite often prompts a full backslide and you should start from the very beginning once more. Try not to think 'only one won't do any harm. It will!

Each day in turn

Focus on breaking to the completion of the day. The principal little while is the hardest, so require each day in turn. This guidance might seem like simply one more banality, yet numerous smokers have found it has a major effect on stopping effectively or not.

It means a lot to prepare, yet don't stress over how you will adapt at the workplace Christmas celebration toward the year's end.

Desires and withdrawal side effects

Assuming you are taking quit-smoking medicine, the desires and withdrawal side effects ought to be reasonable. Assuming that they are irksome, your prescription might should be changed.

Desires just last 2-3 minutes, albeit that might feel like until the end of time! Divert yourself by thinking or accomplishing something different and they will pass. Desires get more vulnerable and less regular after some time however can keep going for a long time.

Nicotine withdrawal side effects are brief and for the most part, settle within two or three weeks as your body changes. It is useful to see these as recuperation side effects, an indication of the body mending itself.

Normal withdrawal side effects are

Touchiness, disappointment, animosity

Expanded craving and weight gain (will in general be enduring)
Trouble concentrating
Anxiety
Discouraged mind-set
Upset rest
Different impacts of stopping

Hack or sore throat in the main weeks in the wake of stopping
Mouth ulcers
Stoppage
Keep occupied and dynamic
You will have additional free time when you quit and keeping occupied will assist with diverting you from pondering cigarettes. It might assist with making a rundown of exercises you could do when you are feeling exhausted. Download this rundown of 185 tomfoolery and pleasant exercises to assist with filling the opening which is many times left after stopping.

Remember to routinely work-out. Indeed, even a short 10-minute walk diminishes desires, and withdrawal side effects ease pressure and forestalls weight gain. Attempt to practice as a general rule.

Inspiration card

While hankering strikes, it is not difficult to fail to remember why you are putting yourself through this inconvenience! It can assist with making a rundown of why you need to stop on a little card and haul this around with you. Take out the card when important to remind yourself why stopping is so significant.

Figure out how to say no

Seeing others smoke or being offered a cigarette is a typical reason for returning to smoking. Consequently, it is useful to arrange for how to say no when it occurs as it will happen eventually

Instances of how to reject a cigarette are:

'Forget about it Sway, I don't smoke any longer.'
'Gratitude for offering Kate, yet I quit smoking and don't have any desire to smoke at any point down the road.'
'Pass Pete, I'm a non-smoker now.'
What on the off chance that you slip?
Sneaks through the main little while are for the most part because of nicotine withdrawal and might be an indication that you want more medicine.

If you have a slip, don't whip yourself! Nothing surprising. The significant thing is to refocus quickly to try not to slip into a full backslide.

A slip is an important growth opportunity. For what reason did it happen? How might you manage what is happening assuming that it emerges once more?

On the off chance that you are on quit smoking drug, keeping on taking it after a slip is significant. Keep your nicotine fix on and keep on taking your tablets or other treatment. Your prescription will assist you with gaining back influence in the future.

Caffeine and liquor

Make sure to lessen your caffeine, as a rule by about a half. Scale back your drinking likewise makes stopping more straightforward.

Long haul Techniques

Be careful with arrogance

Following half a month, you are getting along nicely and feeling certain. That is perfect, yet don't get pompous! A great many people backslide even at this stage.

Desires

It's generally expected to keep on getting desires in circumstances in which you used to smoke. Having 'only one cigarette' could mean starting from the very beginning once more. Remain watchful and mindful of the gamble.

Keep speedy acting NRT convenient

Convey a fast-acting type of nicotine (mouth splash, capsule, gum, inhalator) with you consistently. On the off chance that you are hit with a surprising desire to smoke, a portion of speedy-acting nicotine can give help. The mouth shower is the quickest-acting item and begins to assuage desires following 60 seconds. On the off chance that is conceivable, expect desires and have a portion of nicotine 15-20 minutes in advance.

Continue to take your medicine

It is enticing to stop your medicine when things are working out in a good way. Perhaps you don't require it any longer. Notwithstanding, the drug is one reason you are getting along nicely, and halting it rashly will diminish your likelihood of coming out on top. It will likewise give you assurance against abrupt and unforeseen desires. Ensure you proceed with your medicine for a full course, no less than 8-12 weeks.

Be careful with allurements

The normal reasons for backsliding after the initial not many weeks are:

Stress or profound surprise

Liquor

Being around different smokers

It is indispensable to know about these triggers, to design procedures to manage them or even to keep away from them on the off chance that fundamental until you feel somewhat more grounded. The most compelling thing is to refocus as soon as could be expected. Consider how far you have come. It would be such a disgrace to need to go through the entire shopping process once more.

Your way of life

Remember to keep yourself involved and keep a sound way of life. Is it true or not that you are practicing more according to plan? Practicing after you quit has been displayed to diminish the gamble of backsliding. It likewise assists with diminishing pressure and controlling weight gain. Is it true or not that you are rehearsing your pressure decrease systems? Is it safe to say that you are getting a charge out of new without smoke exercises and interests which keep you involved and stop you from contemplating cigarettes?

Nicotine Withdrawal Course of events

The greater part of these side effects will top during the second or the third day into the end cycle. Not every person who quits smoking will encounter every one of them a great many people will have the hardest time battling desires, peevishness, and challenging thinking so they probably won't see the rest.

The initial 72 hours are the most horrendously terrible for most smokers so how about we center around them?

4 hours after a cigarette - Your body is flagging that it's the ideal opportunity for a cigarette. Nicotine in your framework has dropped by 90 % and you will begin filling nervous. This is the point at which the hankering begins. Rather than respecting enticement, take a stab at zeroing in on something different - clean the house, iron every one of your shirts, or go out for a run. The desire for nicotine will pass yet you should prepare yourselves for when it begins once more.

10 hours after a cigarette - You as of now have various desire episodes behind you yet now is the ideal time to prepare for bed. Certain individuals will begin encountering strange cravings right now - this is because your glucose levels are lower than expected and encountering hunger in this period is normal. You could likewise begin feeling a

shivering sensation in your grasp and feet - flow is getting back to business as usual and it's not something to be frightened by. Drink a lot of water, wrap yourself up and get ready to brave it. Most smokers cave as of now - it's more straightforward to smoke a cigarette than to confront a restless evening. Fundamentally, you lock in - after this obstacle, every night without a cigarette will be more straightforward.

24 hours after a cigarette - This will an extreme stir. Contingent upon your smoking propensities you could get a desire to light a cigarette when you open your eyes. Battle it. Have something to eat and drink a lot of liquids - stay away from espresso, tea, or whatever other refreshment that could act as a trigger. It's likewise essential to allow yourself to handle everything. You will probably be touchy and restless - this is because your body is running on 0 nicotine as of now. Attempt to begin another daily practice. Run, weave, compose, or do

anything more that is not difficult to do once you get an inclination to light a cigarette.

48 hours following a cigarette - One day left and the most terrible is finished. As of now, you could begin encountering discouragement or nervousness - all typical as your cerebrum science begins to get acclimated to the absence of nicotine. Migraines may be a slight issue however these ought to disappear in the following 24 hours. Desires are as yet consistent and somebody who was a typical smoker will insight something like 4-6 episodes each day. Help yourself to remember why you're doing this and have your option on backup assuming the desires get too challenging to even consider making due (wear your running stuff to work, have a journal prepared, and keep that chunk of yarn and your needles close).

72 hours after a cigarette - Desires are dying down impressively and their span time shouldn't surpass five minutes for each episode. Engage your psyche during those 5

minutes and involve yourself with some different options from pondering a cigarette and desires will die down. Certain individuals, particularly weighty smokers, could encounter an irritated throat and inordinate hacking. This is because your body is freeing itself of tar covering and developing new tissue. This is frequently joined by snugness in the chest that is brought about by hacking.

7 - 21 days - Periodic desires for nicotine strike consistently yet they are sensible generally. It's critical to perceive the truth about them and to advise yourselves that lighting a cigarette wouldn't just exacerbate the situation, it would hinder you impressively - back to the starting point, to be precise. A great many people notice that their craving is expanded however their degrees of energy appear to be lower. Assuming it happens to you this is because your digestion is starting to standardize and your glucose levels are dropping. Both tooting and stoppage could happen because

gastrointestinal developments are additionally dialing back.
Over 70% of smokers who choose to stop will encounter nicotine desires and expanded hunger.

Around 60% of individuals will experience the ill effects of uneasiness, despondency, unfortunate focus, or peevishness - these psychological side effects can endure as long as about a month but will slowly die down. Assuming they persevere, we encourage you to converse with your PCP about them.

Helped Suspension
The situation portrayed above applies to smokers who choose to stop without help. Help, in this situation, implies nicotine substitution treatment. Not every person has the endurance or self-discipline to go through one or the other's entirely okay. Still up in the air to stop the propensity have a ton of nicotine substitution choices available to them. Assuming that you choose

to utilize them ensure you work it out with your PCP and adhere to the directions.

Side effects of nicotine withdrawal won't be so conspicuous on the off chance that your body is getting nicotine from sources other than a cigarette. NTR ought to be utilized on a case-by-case basis as there is a risk of subbing one habit with another. Following 8 to 12 weeks you ought to begin bringing down the portion of nicotine you are managing to yourself until you're total without nicotine.

www.ingramcontent.com/pod-product-compliance
Lightning Source LLC
LaVergne TN
LVHW052046160826
845678LV00015B/3126

9798362402570